I0427401

KIDNEY DIALYSIS

DIET

COOKBOOK

FOR BEGINNERS

The Ultimate Guide with 20 Delicious & Quick Recipes for helping Dialysis Patients manage Kidney Disease

Patricia Camire

CHECK OTHER BOOKS BY AUTHOR:

TABLE OF CONTENT

INTRODUCTION

Meet Sarah, a determined person navigating the tricky waters of renal illness. Sarah was intimidated when her doctor explained the prospect of renal dialysis, but tenacity propelled her forward.

Patricia Camire's "Kidney Dialysis Diet Cookbook for Beginners" changed Sarah's perspective on limited diets.

Sarah flicked through the cookbook's pages, discovering a world where kidney-friendly foods were not only nutritional but also flavorful.

The meticulously developed meals gave a road map to a tasty diet while also balanced renal health.

From inventive breakfast selections to delectable desserts, each dish provided an occasion for Sarah to embrace life.

The cookbook not only addressed food issues, but it also provided a sense of empowerment.

Sarah found delight in the kitchen, cooking meals that were both nutritious and tasty.

The anxiety of boring, repetitive meals dissipated, giving way to a renewed appreciation for the cookbook's various and pleasant flavors.

Sarah's adventure with the "Kidney Dialysis Diet Cookbook" was more than just about managing her health; it was also a celebration of culinary exploration, demonstrating that a kidney-friendly diet can be a delicious trip, one recipe at a time.

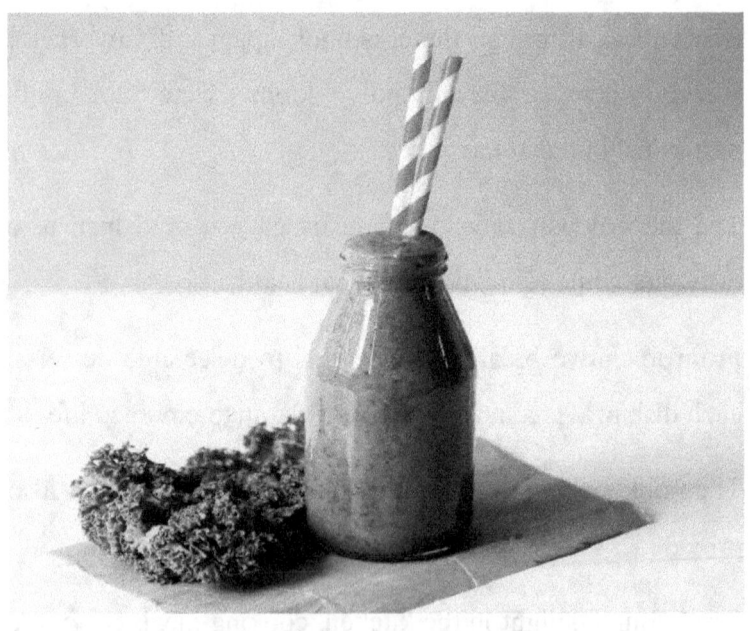

CHAPTER ONE

UNDERSTANDING KIDNEY DIALYSIS AND ITS DIETARY IMPLICATIONS

Kidney dialysis is a life-saving medical used to manage renal disease. The purpose of hemodialysis, which utilizes a machine to filter the blood, and peritoneal dialysis, which uses the lining of the abdomen to do the same, is to eliminate waste and excess fluids from the body. Understanding the fundamentals of dialysis is the first step toward successful management of renal disease.

Types of Dialysis

1. **Hemodialysis**:

   - Involves an artificial kidney machine (dialyzer) to filter the blood.

   - Usually executed in a dialysis center.

   - Sessions typically run around four hours and are held multiple times each week.

2. Peritoneal Dialysis:

- Uses the peritoneum as a natural filter.

- Can be performed from home, offering greater flexibility.

- Involves the exchange of fluids via a catheter, which is normally done daily.

Dietary Challenges for Dialysis Patients

Living with renal illness creates dietary issues since the kidneys' reduced function impairs the body's capacity to metabolize certain nutrients.

Dialysis, while necessary for controlling the disease, complicates dietary requirements.

Restrictions on Nutrients

1. Fluid Intake:

- Limiting fluid intake is essential to avoid fluid overload, a typical problem for dialysis patients.

- Monitoring and managing fluid consumption becomes a daily requirement.

2. Sodium (Salt):

- Kidney illness often leads to sodium retention.

- Strict sodium management is required to maintain blood pressure and fluid balance.

3. Potassium:

- Impaired kidneys struggle to control potassium levels.

- Dialysis patients should avoid high-potassium meals to avoid problems.

4. Phosphorus:

- Kidney disease might lead to elevated phosphorus levels.

- Dietary management includes minimizing phosphorus-rich foods.

5. Protein:

- Protein requirements may differ for dialysis patients.

- Maintaining a balanced protein intake is critical for preventing malnutrition without overburdening the kidneys.

Importance of Managing Protein Intake

While protein is necessary for overall health, too much protein can strain the kidneys. Dialysis patients frequently have to find a fine balance between getting enough protein for energy and muscle maintenance and without overloading their kidneys.

To traverse the complexities of a kidney-friendly diet, it is critical to understand the nutritional requirements.

The emphasis is not just on restriction, but also on ensuring that the body obtains the necessary nutrients in the proper proportions.

Key Nutrients for Dialysis Patients

1. Protein:

- Essential for maintaining muscle mass.

- Lean meats, poultry, fish, eggs, and plant-based foods are all possible sources.

2. Vitamins:

- Adequate consumption of vitamins B and C is necessary.

- Balanced meals that include a range of fruits and vegetables help to meet vitamin requirements.

3. Minerals:

- Monitor potassium and phosphorus levels regularly.

- Selecting low-potassium and low-phosphorus meals aids in maintaining equilibrium.

Guidelines for Maintaining a Balanced Diet

1. Individualized Dietary Plans:

- Collaborating with healthcare providers to develop customized diet regimens.

- Taking into consideration personal health, interests, and lifestyle.

2. Balancing Act:

- Finding a balance between nutritional needs and restrictions.

- Trying out different cooking methods and ingredients.

3. Supplements:

- Assessing the necessity for supplements to fulfill particular nutrient needs.

- Collaborating with healthcare providers to assess supplement need.

Building a Foundation for Kidney-Friendly Eating

Practical parts of following a kidney-friendly diet include daily decisions about grocery shopping, meal preparation, and portion management.

Building a foundation for kidney-friendly diet entails not just what to eat but also how to make educated decisions.

Tips for Grocery Shopping

1. Reading Food Labels:

- Developing the skill of reading food labels to identify sodium, potassium, and phosphorus content.

- Selecting packaged meals with lower amounts of these minerals.

2. Fresh Produce Choices:

- Opting for fresh fruits and vegetables, considering their nutrient content and lower processing.

Kitchen Practices for Meal Preparation

1. Cooking Techniques:

- Discovering ways to increase taste without using too much salt.

- Using herbs, spices, and other condiments to enhance flavor.

2. Portion Control:

- Recognize the significance of portion management in regulating nutritional intake.

- Avoiding excessive consumption of potassium or phosphorus-rich meals.

Addressing Common Concerns and Myths

Navigating a kidney-friendly diet typically raises similar worries and misconceptions.

Addressing these challenges front on allows people to accept their nutritional journey constructively.

1. Taste and Variety:

  - Dispelling the idea that a kidney-friendly diet is bland and lacks variety.

  - Featuring different meals that are palatable while adhering to dietary restrictions.

2. Satisfaction in Restricted Diets:

  - Emphasizing the necessity of having fulfilling meals despite dietary constraints.

  - Promoting a good attitude towards culinary inquiry and innovation.

Understanding renal dialysis and its nutritional consequences is critical for those treating kidney illness.

This chapter has provided the framework by discussing the various forms of dialysis, the obstacles that dialysis patients confront, and the nutritional requirements for their well-being.

Moving forward, the Kidney Dialysis Diet Cookbook will dig into practical recipes and suggestions to make the transition to kidney-friendly diet fun and rewarding.

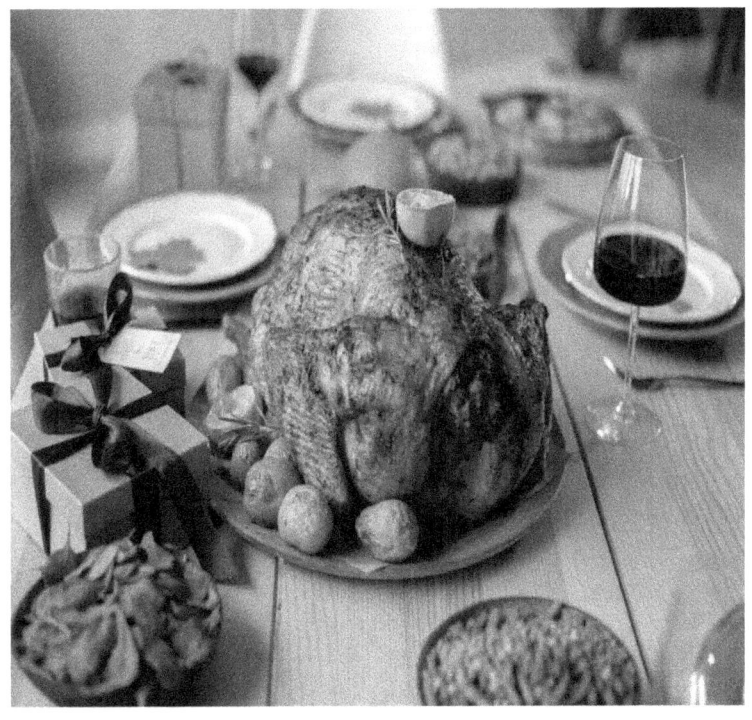

CHAPTER TWO

DELICIOUS & QUICK KIDNEY DIALYSIS DIET RECIPES

1. Grilled Lemon Herb Chicken

Ingredients:

- 4 boneless and skinless chicken breasts

- Two teaspoons of olive oil

- 1 juiced lemon

- 2 chopped garlic cloves

- 1 teaspoon of dried oregano

- Add Salt and pepper to taste

Prep Time: 15 minutes

Cook Time: 20 minutes

Serves: 4

Instructions:

1. In a mixing bowl, combine olive oil, lemon juice, minced garlic, dried oregano, salt, and pepper to make the marinade.

2. Place the chicken breasts in a resealable plastic bag, add the marinade, and refrigerate for at least an hour.

3. Preheat the grill to medium-high.

4. Grill the chicken for 8-10 minutes per side, or until well done.

5. Serve over steamed veggies or a kidney-friendly salad.

2. Quinoa and Vegetable Stir-Fry

Ingredients:

- 1 cup of quinoa

- Two glasses of water

- Two teaspoons of olive oil

- 1 sliced onion

- 2 sliced bell peppers

- 1 sliced zucchini

- 2 julienned carrots

- 2 minced garlic cloves

- 3 tablespoons of low-sodium soy sauce

Prep Time: 15 minutes

Cook Time: 20 minutes

Serves: 4

Instructions:

1. Rinse the quinoa under cold water and cook according per package directions.

2. In a large pan, increase the olive oil temperature over medium heat. Add the chopped onion, bell peppers, zucchini, carrots, and minced garlic.

3. Stir-fry the veggies until they are soft and crunchy.

4. Pour soy sauce over the cooked quinoa in the pan. Stir well to mix.

5. Cook for an extra 5 minutes to ensure that everything is well heated.

6. Serve warm for a healthy and kidney-friendly stir-fry.

3. Berry and Spinach Smoothie

Ingredients:

- One cup of fresh spinach leaves

- ½ cup of mixed berries (strawberries, blueberries, raspberries)

- 1 banana

- ½ cup of low-fat yogurt

- 1 tablespoon of chia seeds

- 1 cup of water or almond milk

- Ice cubes (optional)

Prep Time: 5 minutes

Serves: 2

Instructions:

1. In a blender, combine fresh spinach, mixed berries, banana, low-fat yogurt, chia seeds, and water (or almond milk).

2. Blend until smooth and creamy. If you like a cooler consistency, add some ice cubes.

3. Pour the smoothie into glasses and enjoy this delicious and kidney-friendly beverage.

4. Lemon Dill Baked Salmon

Ingredients:

- 4 salmon fillets

- 2 teaspoons of olive oil

- One lemon, zested and juiced

- 2 tablespoons fresh dill, chopped

- Add Salt and pepper to taste

Prep Time: 10 minutes

Cook Time: 15 minutes

Serves: 4

Instructions:

1. Preheat your oven to 400°F (200°C).

2. Arrange the salmon fillets on a baking pan lined with parchment paper.

3. In a small mixing bowl, combine olive oil, lemon zest, lemon juice, chopped dill, salt, and pepper to make the marinade.

4. Brush the marinade onto each salmon fillet.

5. Bake in the preheated oven for 12-15 minutes, or until the salmon is well cooked.

5. Mediterranean Quinoa Salad

Ingredients:

- 1 cup of cooked quinoa

- 1 diced cucumber

- 1 cup of halved cherry tomatoes

- ½ cup of Kalamata olives, pitted and sliced

- ¼ cup of feta cheese, crumbled

- Two teaspoons of extra-virgin olive oil

- One tablespoon of red wine vinegar

- Fresh basil leaves (optional as garnish)

Prep Time: 15 minutes

Serves: 4

Instructions:

1. In a large mixing bowl, add cooked quinoa, chopped cucumber, cherry tomatoes, sliced Kalamata olives, and crumbled feta cheese.

2. In a small dish, combine olive oil and red wine vinegar. Pour the salad with the dressing until well combined.

3. Optional: garnish with fresh basil leaves.

4. Refrigerate for a cold salad.

6. Roasted Vegetable Hummus Wrap

Ingredients:

- Whole-grain wraps
- 1 cup of hummus
- 1 sliced zucchini
- 1 sliced bell pepper
- 1 sliced red onion
- 1 tablespoon of olive oil
- 1 teaspoon of cumin
- Add Salt and pepper to taste

Prep Time: 20 minutes

Cook Time: 15 minutes

Serves: 4

Instructions:

1. Preheat oven to 425°F (220°C).

2. Toss the sliced zucchini, bell pepper, and red onion with olive oil, cumin, salt, and pepper.

3. Roast the veggies in the preheated oven for 15 minutes, or until soft.

4. Spread hummus over whole grain wrappers and top with roasted veggies.

5. Roll up the wraps and serve for a hearty, kidney-friendly lunch.

7. Baked Eggplant Parmesan

Ingredients:

- 1 big sliced eggplant

- 1 cup of whole-grain breadcrumbs

- ½ cup of grated Parmesan cheese

- One teaspoon of dried oregano

- One teaspoon of dried basil

- 2 cups of low-sodium marinara sauce

- 1 cup of part-skim mozzarella cheese, shredded

Prep Time: 20 minutes

Cook Time: 25 minutes

Serves: 4

Instructions:

1. Preheat your oven to 400°F (200°C).

2. Coat the eggplant slices in whole-grain breadcrumbs seasoned with dried oregano, basil, and Parmesan cheese.

3. Transfer the oiled eggplant slices to a baking sheet and bake for 15-20 minutes, or until golden brown.

4. In a baking dish, combine baked eggplant pieces, marinara sauce, and shredded mozzarella.

5. Bake in the oven until the cheese is melted and bubbling.

8. Cilantro-Lime Shrimp Tacos

Ingredients:

- 1 pound of peeled and deveined shrimp

- 2 tablespoons of olive oil

- 2 juiced limes

- ¼ cup of chopped fresh cilantro

- 1 teaspoon of cumin

- Whole-grain tortillas

- Shredded cabbage and salsa for topping

Prep Time: 15 minutes

Cook Time: 5 minutes

Serves: 4

Instructions:

1. In a bowl, combine the shrimp, olive oil, lime juice, chopped cilantro, and cumin.

2. Cook the shrimp in a pan over medium heat for 2-3 minutes per side, or until completely done.

3. Warm whole-grain tortillas and fill them with cooked shrimp, chopped cabbage, and salsa.

9. Greek Salad with Lemon Herb Dressing

Ingredients:

- 4 cups of mixed salad greens

- 1 sliced cucumber

- 1 cup of halved cherry tomatoes

- ½ of sliced red onion

- ½ cup of crumbled feta cheese

- 2 tablespoons of olive oil

- 1 lemon (juiced)

- 1 teaspoon of dried oregano

- Add Salt and pepper to taste

Prep Time: 15 minutes

Serves: 4

Instructions:

1. In a large mixing bowl, add salad greens, sliced cucumber, cherry tomatoes, red onion, and crumbled feta cheese.

2. In a small mixing bowl, combine olive oil, lemon juice, dried oregano, salt, and pepper to make the dressing.

3. Drizzle the salad with the dressing and gently toss to coat.

10. Turkey and Vegetable Skewers

Ingredients:

- 1 pound of turkey breast (cut into chunks)

- 1 sliced zucchini

- 1 chopped bell pepper

- Cherry tomatoes

- Add 2 tablespoons of olive oil

- 1 teaspoon of garlic powder

- One teaspoon of dried thyme

- Add Salt and pepper to taste

Prep Time: 20 minutes

Cook Time: 15 minutes

Serves: 4

Instructions:

1. Preheat your grill or grill pan.

2. In a mixing dish, add turkey pieces, sliced zucchini, bell pepper chunks, cherry tomatoes, olive oil, garlic powder, dried thyme, salt, and pepper.

3. Thread the turkey and veggie pieces on skewers.

4. Grill the skewers for 12-15 minutes, rotating regularly, until the turkey is well cooked.

11. Cauliflower and Broccoli Stir-Fry

Ingredients:

- 2 cups of cauliflower florets

- 2 cups of broccoli florets

- 1 julienned carrot

- 2 tablespoons of low-sodium soy sauce

- One tablespoon of sesame oil

- 1 teaspoon of chopped ginger

- 1 minced garlic clove

- 1 tablespoon of rice vinegar

Prep Time: 15 minutes

Cook Time: 10 minutes

Serves: 4

Instructions:

1. Heat the sesame oil in a wok or big pan over medium heat.

2. Stir-fry cauliflower florets, broccoli florets, and julienned carrot for about 5-7 minutes, or until soft and crisp.

3. In a small bowl, combine soy sauce, chopped ginger, garlic, and rice vinegar.

4. Pour the sauce over the veggies and toss to combine. Cook for a another 2–3 minutes.

12. Quinoa-Stuffed Bell Peppers

Ingredients:

- 4 bell peppers, halved and seeds removed

- 1 cup of cooked quinoa

- 1 can of black beans (drained and rinsed)

- 1 cup of corn kernels

- 1 cup of diced tomatoes

- 1 teaspoon of cumin

- 1 teaspoon of chili powder

- ½ cup of grated cheddar cheese (optional)

Prep Time: 25 minutes

Cook Time: 25 minutes

Serves: 4

Instructions:

1. Preheat your oven to 375°F (190°C).

2. In a bowl, combine the cooked quinoa, black beans, corn kernels, chopped tomatoes, cumin, and chili powder.

3. Spoon the quinoa mixture into the halved bell peppers.

4. If wanted, add some shredded cheddar cheese on top.

5. Bake in the oven for 25 minutes, or until the peppers are soft.

13. Lemon Herb Baked Chicken

Ingredients:

- 4 boneless, skinless chicken breasts

- 2 juiced lemons

- 2 tablespoons of olive oil

- 2 teaspoons of dried thyme

- 1 teaspoon of dried rosemary

- 1 teaspoon of garlic powder

- Add Salt and pepper to taste

Prep Time: 15 minutes

Cook Time: 25 minutes

Serves: 4

Instructions:

1. Preheat your oven to 400°F (200°C).

2. In a bowl, combine lemon juice, olive oil, dried thyme, dried rosemary, garlic powder, salt, and pepper.

3. Place the chicken breasts in a baking tray and pour the lemon herb mixture over.

4. Bake for approximately 20-25 minutes, or until the chicken is well done.

14. Spinach and Mushroom Quiche

Ingredients:

- 1 pre-made whole wheat pie crust

- 1 cup of chopped fresh spinach

- 1 cup of sliced mushrooms

- 4 big eggs

- One cup of low-fat milk

- ½ cup of shredded Swiss cheese

- Salt and pepper to taste

Prep Time: 15 minutes

Cook Time: 35 minutes

Serves: 6

Instructions:

1. Preheat oven to 375°F (190°C).

2. In a skillet, cook the chopped spinach and sliced mushrooms until wilted.

3. In a mixing dish, combine eggs, milk, salt, and pepper.

4. Place the pie crust in a pie plate, then add the sautéed veggies, pour the egg mixture over them, and top with shredded Swiss cheese.

5. Bake for approximately 30-35 minutes, or until the quiche is set.

15. Watermelon and Feta Salad

Ingredients:

- 4 cups of sliced seedless watermelon

- 1 cup of chopped cucumber

- ½ cup of crumbled feta cheese

- 2 tablespoons of chopped fresh mint

- One tablespoon of balsamic glaze

Prep Time: 10 minutes

Serves: 4

Instructions:

1. In a large bowl, mix cubed watermelon, chopped cucumber, and crumbled feta cheese.

2. Add fresh mint to the salad.

3. Drizzle with balsamic glaze right before serving

16. Mediterranean Chickpea Salad

Ingredients:

- 1 can of drained and washed chickpeas

- 1 cup of halved cherry tomatoes

- One cucumber, diced

- ½ red onion, finely chopped

- ¼ cup of Kalamata olives, pitted and sliced

- Two teaspoons of extra virgin olive oil

- One tablespoon of red wine vinegar

- One teaspoon of dried oregano

- Add Salt and pepper to taste

Prep Time: 15 minutes

Serves: 4

Instructions:

1. In a large mixing bowl, add chickpeas, cherry tomatoes, diced cucumber, chopped red onion, and sliced Kalamata olives.

2. In a small dish, combine the olive oil, red wine vinegar, dried oregano, salt, and pepper.

3. Pour the dressing over the salad and gently stir. Serve cold.

17. Salmon and Asparagus Foil Packets

Ingredients:

- 4 salmon fillets

- 1 bunch of trimmed asparagus

- 2 tablespoons of lemon juice

- 2 tablespoons of chopped fresh dill

- 1 tablespoon of olive oil

- Add Salt and pepper to taste

Prep Time: 15 minutes

Cook Time: 20 minutes

Serves: 4

Instructions:

1. Preheat your oven to 400°F (200°C).

2. Place one salmon fillet on a piece of foil. Arrange the trimmed asparagus around the fish.

3. Drizzle lemon juice and olive oil on the fish and asparagus. Sprinkle with chopped fresh dill, salt, and pepper.

4. Seal the foil packets and bake for about 20 minutes, or until the salmon is well cooked.

18. Quinoa and Vegetable Stir-Fry

Ingredients:

- 1 cup of cooked quinoa

- 1 cup of broccoli florets

- One sliced bell pepper

- One julienned carrot

- 1 sliced zucchini

- 2 tablespoons of low-sodium soy sauce

- One tablespoon of sesame oil

- Mince 1 teaspoon of ginger

- 1 minced garlic clove

Prep Time: 20 minutes

Cook Time: 15 minutes

Serves: 4

Instructions:

1. Increase the sesame oil temperature in a large pan or wok over medium-high heat.

2. Combine the sliced bell pepper, julienned carrot, sliced zucchini, and broccoli florets. Stir-fry for approximately 5-7 minutes, or until veggies are tender-crisp.

3. Add the cooked quinoa to the veggies.

4. In a small bowl, combine the low-sodium soy sauce, chopped ginger, and garlic. Pour the sauce onto the quinoa and veggies. Stir-fry for another 2-3 minutes.

19. Turkey and Vegetable Skewers

Ingredients:

- 1 pound of turkey breast (cut into cubes)

- 1 sliced zucchini

- 1 sliced yellow bell pepper

- One red onion sliced into bits

- Two teaspoons of olive oil

- One tablespoon of balsamic vinegar

- One teaspoon of dried thyme

- Add Salt and pepper to taste

Prep Time: 20 minutes (plus marinating time)

Cook Time: 15 minutes

Serves: 4

Instructions:

1. In a mixing bowl, combine olive oil, balsamic vinegar, dried thyme, salt, and pepper to make the marinade.

2. Place turkey cubes, zucchini slices, bell pepper slices, and red onion chunks on skewers.

3. Brush the marinade onto the skewers and leave to marinate for at least 30 minutes.

4. Grill the skewers for 15 minutes, or until the turkey is well cooked.

20. Berry and Almond Smoothie Bowl

Ingredients:

- 1 cup of mixed berries such as strawberries, blueberries, and raspberries

- 1 sliced banana

- ½ cup of low-fat yogurt

- ¼ cup of almonds, chopped

- 1 tablespoon chia seeds

- Honey for drizzling (optional)

Prep Time: 10 minutes

Serves: 2

Instructions:

1. In a blender, combine the mixed berries, sliced banana, and low-fat yogurt. Blend until smooth.

2. Pour the smoothie into bowls.

3. Garnish with chopped almonds, chia seeds, and honey if preferred.

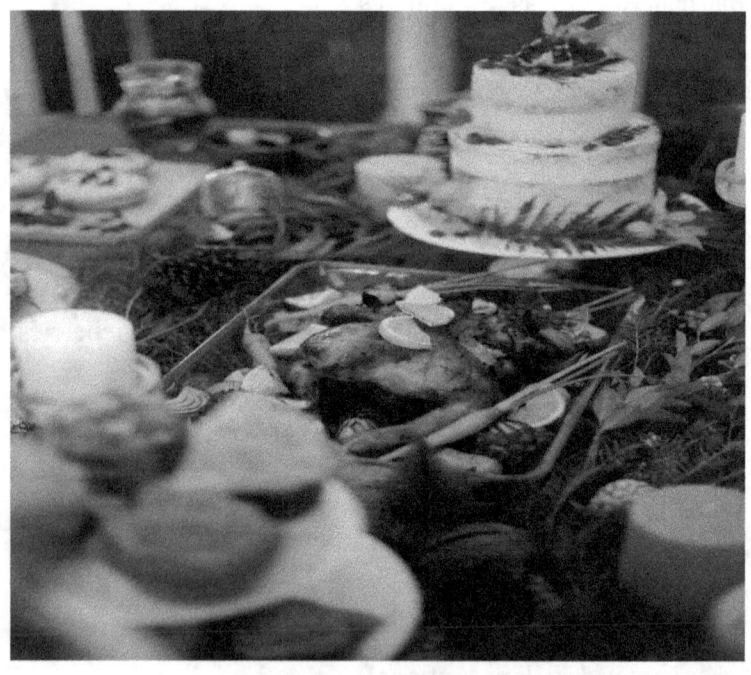

CONCLUSION

Patricia Camire provides more than simply recipes in the last chapters of the "Kidney Dialysis Diet Cookbook for Beginners," imparting a culinary philosophy that transcends dietary constraints.

Chapter One establishes the groundwork, providing insights and practical advice for managing renal health gracefully.

As you work your way through the scrumptious dishes, each one demonstrates the perfect balance of flavor and kidney-friendly nutrients.

This cookbook is more than simply a list of things to avoid; it is also a celebration of what may be enjoyed. Camire's recipes inspire you to adopt a lifestyle that feeds both your body and your spirit.

As the book concludes, it leaves a tasty legacy—an encouragement to savor every meal on the road to kidney health and general well-being.

As you flip the final page of the "Kidney Dialysis Diet Cookbook for Beginners," please accept my deepest thanks.

It has been an honor to share this culinary journey with you—one distinguished by delectable food, conscious decisions, and a dedication to renal health.

Thank you for welcoming me into your kitchens and adopting a lifestyle that balances nutrition and taste. May each meal bring delight to your table and improve your well-being.

Remember, this is more than just a cookbook; it's a culinary partner on your search for a healthy, kidney-friendly lifestyle. Here's to enjoying excellent health, one tasty recipe at a time.

With gratitude,

Patricia Camire

HAPPY COOKING!